Bitten

A Tick Survivor's Warning About the Growing Tick Crisis

Don't Brush It Off

Jennifer Saterdal

Published by Don't Brush It Off Publishing An imprint of NextJen LLC Puyallup, Washington

jennifersaterdal.com

This book is based on personal experience and is not intended to provide medical advice. Always consult a qualified healthcare provider regarding any medical concerns.

All factual information has been researched to the best of the author's ability. Sources are listed in the Resources and Sources section.

ISBN 979-8-9881520-0-2

Dedication

For my mom and my grandma. You always said someone should write about this.

Mom, you held it together when everything fell apart at once. You got us through it.

Love, Jennifer

Grandma, who knew your magazine subscriptions would end up saving our lives? Best investment you ever made.

Love, Jenny

The breakthrough is usually one crazy lady away!

-Jennifer Saterdal

Table of Contents

A Note Before You Begin

This book has been a long time coming.

It started years ago when I overheard my mother and grandmother talking about that stretch of time in Florida. How insane it was. How much happened at once and how someone should write a book about it.

I never forgot that conversation.

Before I tell you, what happened that summer, I want to tell you about my grandmother. Her name was Beverly. She had big-spirited energy and a cigarette-stained laugh that filled whatever room she was in. She dyed her hair shades of red her whole life, and she pulled it off completely. Not everyone can do that, but she could. Some say similar to Lucille Ball, even.

She was the only person in the world allowed to call me Jenny. My mother had strong feelings about that nickname. Beverly called me Jenny anyway. I always wondered if she did it partly just to get under my mom's skin.

When my little brother Sal and I were sick in that Florida hospital, she played cards with me as I got better and brought us little Dachshund puppets. I still have mine in a bin in the garage. I have never been able to get rid of it.

My grandma was a secretary and she raised four children. Life was not easy on her, and she deserved better than some of what it handed her. But she showed up for us. That is what I remember most. Grandma showed up.

She is one of the reasons this book exists. The other is that tick awareness needs more attention than it's getting, and it could save lives. I feel it's my duty. See something, say something. As the saying goes.

My life has taught me that bad luck doesn't always come in threes, the way people say. For me, it comes in what I now call shit streaks. Long ones. And that summer in Florida was my first.

I originally planned for this story to be a chapter in a larger memoir. I didn't think it could stand alone. But as I watched the headlines change, as tick-borne illnesses kept rising, as a Congressional investigation opened into whether the government had weaponized ticks, and as the first person died from a tick bite that made them allergic to red meat, I went back to that chapter and looked at it differently.

It could stand alone. It should stand alone.

People need this information. And I need to be the one to share it, because I have lived it in a way most people haven't. I survived something that should have killed me. I have paid attention my whole life because life taught me early what happens when you don't.

This is not a medical textbook. It is a true story with facts attached. My hope is that somewhere in these pages you find something that helps you, protects someone you love, or simply makes you feel less alone in whatever you are navigating.

Every year, an estimated 31 million Americans are bitten by a tick. That is nearly one in ten people. Reported cases of tick-borne disease have more than doubled in the past two decades. And most people still don't know what ticks are carrying.

Pay attention. Don't brush it off.

Chapter 1:

The Day of the Doberman

Before the tick, there was a dog. This is where the story really starts.

It was a Saturday night, back in 1979. I was three years old. Sal was one and a half. My parents had dropped us off at a sitter's for a date night.

Unbeknownst to everyone, the sitter's neighbor had a tall black Doberman with golden brown accents. You know, the typical Doberman markings. According to my mom, the owner allegedly had the dog locked in a room without food or water for an undisclosed amount of time. It must have been a long time for it to get itself out of the room. You would think it would have had to pretty much eat the door, to get out. Anyway, at some point, the dog made its way out of the room, through its owner's home, and into the sitter's house and I was the first thing he saw.

I never even saw him coming.

The dog grabbed me by the back of the neck. His teeth pierced my skin and he shook me. My feet flew up off the ground as he flung me around like I was a rag doll, exposing my spinal cord. The sitter came running in when I screamed. She grabbed for him; he released my neck only to bite it again. It didn't stop. It lunged again, this time sinking his teeth into my right shoulder. Then the back of my right calf. By the time she finally wrestled his raging body away from mine I had fallen onto the carpet. I was bleeding in three places, and I never saw any of it coming. She called 911. Then they called around trying to reach my parents. There were no cell phones back then and the hospital could not do anything without my parents' written consent. So, I waited.

I don't know how long I was there before they arrived. I was three years old, and time doesn't work right at that age, even when nothing terrible is happening. When you are bleeding and frightened and alone in a strange place, time stops meaning anything at all. I remember the carpet. I remember the sounds. I remember people moving around me with urgency and trying to keep their voices calm at the same time. Children always hear the urgency underneath.

What I know from being told is that the sitter stayed with me the entire time. She did not leave my side. She held my hand. She talked to me. Unfortunately, I don't remember her face or her name, and I have never been able to find out who she was.

I was told the sitter acted quickly and didn't freeze. Thankfully, she got the dog off me before it was too late. One centimeter over, according to the doctor, and my spinal cord would have been severed. I may not know her name, but I sure hope she has had a blessed life and that she knows she is a hero. She was heaven-sent. She saved my life that day.

* * *

As my mother tells it, my dad drove through ditches and ran through red lights to get there that day. The message they had received was vague. "Jennifer has been attacked by a Doberman. She needs surgery and they can't do anything without your written consent. They need you here." They really didn't know what they were walking into. They really didn't know what they were about to face.

My dad is a man you notice when he walks into a room. He had shoulder-length, thick, dark brown hair with a wave to it and brown eyes. He sported his bell-bottoms, his black boots, a three-quarter sleeve T-shirt, and his signature wallet with a chain going to his belt. He walked with a certain swagger. His shoulders were back, and his head held high. I could spot that walk anywhere. He loved cars, was an avid fisherman, and would take us snowmobile riding and shanty fishing on the lake sometimes in the winter when we were little. Fishing shanties are so small inside that I landed my butt in the hole of one. My dad was not happy that we had to go back home. It wasn't a far walk but still. I could get hypothermia. He insisted. I can still see the lake frozen over and fishing shanties scattered across it, for what looked like miles.

He came from a big family. His parents were Salvatore Senior and Julie. Everyone called my grandfather Sam, and nobody seems to know why, including people who knew him his whole life. It is one of those family mysteries that I will probably never solve.

They had seven children, all boys except for my Aunt Julie. My grandfather worked for the city doing road work. My grandmother was a stay-at-home mom for most of her life, though she did work at a belt buckle plant for a while. They had a beautiful home in Mount Clemens, Michigan, and two vacation cabins. I recall time at the one in Lapeer fondly. We would walk down to the water and swim around my grandma's ankles. Here is also where I learned about false teeth. Let's just say I was very surprised!

My grandparents prided themselves on being Italian. They had a family tradition of spaghetti dinner every Sunday, and it was an all-must-attend event. Even though I was little, I still remember a full house of people, the guys wrapping each other up in headlocks and giving each other dead legs, and the smell of spaghetti in the air. I can still see my grandma standing at the stove in her orange-and-brown smock apron, stirring her potatoes and meatballs as they simmer in the sauce. She marinated them in it all day. I have never found anything that tasted quite like it since.

I spent a lot of time with my grandparents as a child. I must have because kids usually can't recall the early years the way I do, and I remember so much about their house. The wallpaper looked like old newspapers with clocks, eagles, yarn wheels, and wagons. My grandma kept old bread in the bottom drawer of the oven, and the water always smelled like rotten eggs. I also remember the swing my grandpa built out of wood and a Mary statue in the flower bed just before the garden. I always admired her, and I still couldn't tell you exactly why, but I got myself a smaller one from a garage sale a few years ago. Both of my grandmas would be proud of the deal I got.

We used to hide behind the couch, waiting for grandpa to get home from work so we could jump up and scare him. We'd wait for the screen door and then the doorknob and then jump up and yell. His eyes would get big, and he'd put his hand on his chest and lean back in feigned fright. "Oh, you scared me. I didn't know you were here." And we would laugh.

I also remember the nights when grandpa and I would watch the lightning storms through the screen door while lying on the couch. I remember his hairy chest and how it tickled my cheek and how he made me feel safe. The thunderstorms were beautiful bolts of bright white and yellow, and sometimes a flash of blue, and the crash of thunder would shake me, but I wasn't scared. Not lying there with him.

Unfortunately, my grandmother died of a brain aneurysm when I was in kindergarten. All these years later, I still have never had toast that tasted like hers. She would make ours with butter and give us a glass of milk, then make hers with a hot cup of coffee. Her coffee always smelled so good that I would hound her for a sip. She always said no, it will stunt your growth. Sometimes when she would leave the room, I would take a sip anyway. Every single time, I didn't like it. The smell always fooled me. Call me a slow learner, I guess.

Some people you only know for a few years, and they still leave a mark on you that nothing erases. My grandparents are those people for me. My grandfather was there the night everything happened.

Luckily, surgery had went well and I did not need to have a blood transfusion. I just needed to rest and to let the healing begin.

There had been reporters outside. Word had gotten out about the dog attack somehow. So, when it was time to go, they took us out the back. My mom was carrying me and as we moved through that back exit, she handed me to my grandfather for a moment, and that was when everything that had been held in check finally caught up with her.

It never made the news. We went out the back, and we went home, and that was that.

* * *

A little while later, we met with a lawyer. I remember going into a tall building with huge shiny windows. The front door had a big spinning door, and it took me a moment to want to go through it. I had never seen a skyscraper before. Inside, the lawyer took pictures of my scars. I stood there silently while my mom held up my hair and led them to each one, from my neck to my shoulder to my arm to the back of my leg. Then we were done.

The lawyer's visit didn't result into anything, but the dog was put down. The neighbor faced no consequences that I know of either. A lot of balls were dropped here. And I think about that sometimes, not because of what I lost, but because of what it says about accountability. When you own a powerful animal, you own the consequences of that animal's actions. Full stop. That little girl on the floor deserved better. So do all the children who come after her.

I don't remember most of those days. I was three and a half years old, and my body was in shock. What I remember is the pink and blue toy phones my brother and I received. The tubes running from my neck to my shoulder meant I had to sit still.

* * *

Someone along the way suggested that getting a puppy would help. The idea was that bringing a dog into our lives would keep us from being afraid of them. So, my parents thought it was worth a try.

They brought one home a few months later.

My brother and I screamed. We cried. We climbed directly onto the kitchen table, and we did not come down. We were so distraught and so committed to staying on that table that the puppy did not stay. That wasn't the last dog to join our family, though. I am happy to report that I have had dogs my whole life, and I love them. However, every once in a while, a dog will set something off in me, and I get spooked. I don't take much credit for that reaction though. I think it's the dog that's off, and I can sense it. Bodies remember things the mind lets go of.

I think about that dog sometimes. Not with anger, not anymore. More with a kind of clarity. Animals are honest in a way people aren't. They tell you exactly who they are. The Doberman wasn't evil. He was a large, powerful dog who had been put in a situation he couldn't handle, and he reacted the only way he knew how. What was wrong was that nobody was protecting the dog from its owner or protecting others from the dog. Nobody had thought through what could happen and when it did happen, there were no consequences for anyone except the dog and the child.

That pattern, nobody thinking through what could happen, nobody making sure the right people were held accountable, and the children paying the price for adult oversights. I have seen it enough times in my life that it has become something that I watch for. It is part of why I write notes before doctor appointments. Part of why I push for answers. Part of why I wrote this book.

The world is full of things that can hurt you, that someone else knew about and didn't tell you. Some of those things bite, and some of them are in the grass. I would rather be the person who is too careful than the person who finds out the hard way that nobody was paying attention.

I will say, I still don't care for Dobermans.

A few years ago, I was visiting my dad in Florida, and we went to my stepbrother's house. He had Dobermans of various sizes. When I walked in, they surrounded me as we stood in the dining area of the kitchen. All of them were barking, and everyone in the room went quiet and watched, almost as if to see my reaction. My dad let it go on for a moment, and then he said, without much room for argument: "That's enough. Get them."

I held my composure, but inside I was a little shaken. Not a lot, but it got my attention.

Chapter 2:

The Tick

Before I take you inside that hospital, I want to tell you about my mother.

Her name is Carolyn. She was born in 1958. She is pretty and has always been a hard worker. My mom is a small, petite woman, five foot two, with blue eyes that can light up a room or put the fear of God into you in one quick glance. I got my eyes from her. She has always been a sharp dresser and someone who takes life by the throat and doesn't let go. She worked multiple jobs when she had to, and she never had to be asked. When I was young, she cut hair and then over the years, she did jobs that ranged from cleaning hospital rooms to spot welding. She was a go-getter, and I think I got that partially from her.

She grew up in Detroit in the sixties; she was rough around the edges by necessity. When she talks about those years, she doesn't sugarcoat it. "We are talking the time of the riots, drugs, kids running the town," she said. After school, they went to the party store, picked up their own dinners, and went home and made them. Her parents were devout Catholics, but Detroit had its own curriculum.

When my mom turned seventeen, her parents divorced and moved out of state. They helped her find a place to stay with a man who was a family friend, but he wanted more than she was prepared to give. She never said exactly what happened, but as a woman, I got the drift. She handled it and kept going. That is what she did. That is what she has always done.

When it was time to have me, she boarded a plane from Detroit to Atlanta, seven months along, to be with her mother, Beverly, for the last stretch of her pregnancy. I can only imagine the sense of uncertainty she must have felt. Eighteen years old and unmarried. Going out of state, away from my dad, to have a baby. But she did it anyway. That is very on brand for her.

As my mom tells it, the plane came to a stop on the runway, and she started to feel a few twinges of pain around her belly. She shook it off, attributing it to sitting for so long and having to use the bathroom. She gathered her black leather purse and her carry-on bag and started toward the exit door.

As she came off the ramp, she saw her mother and Grandpa Ken standing there, and next to them, her father, Ernest. It was the first time both of her parents had been in the same place since the divorce. It was also the first time she was meeting Ken, her mother's new husband, a handsome cowboy with a singing voice that registered right up there with the stars. She was eighteen years old, seven months pregnant, meeting her stepfather for the first time, with her ex-husband standing right next to him.

I can only imagine her stomach sank a little.

She got in Ken's van, and they headed to my grandmother's house. When they pulled up, she went to the restroom. Once she came out, she looked over at my uncle John, and they started talking. She looked down, mid-conversation, then looked up. He said, "Your water just broke." The panic set in. She was not due for two months. Looks like I was in a rush to get here. Still to this day, people comment on the fact that I look like I'm in a hurry, but I prefer to say that I am efficient. Sometimes I think that it's an innate quality that I have but others I think it was the way I was raised. You know what I mean right? Didn't your parents tell you? "Think smarter not harder and to take one trip instead of two as well?" Then there is also the fact that us short girls have to learn to walk fast to keep up, and some of us just got a double or a triple whammy.

Anyway, as I was saying, on the way to Atlanta General Hospital all three of her parents were arguing over who Carolyn would ride with and threatening to withhold help if she chose wrong. She was eighteen years old, in labor, and her parents were making it about themselves.

Three hard pushes with only a nurse by her side, and she had me. Four pounds twelve ounces. Not bad for being so early.

Here is the kicker: she went roller skating with my uncle John the day after she was released from the hospital.

I am a mother of three and when I had my first child, I was in labor for thirty-two hours and could barely walk for days. She pushed out a four-pounder and got back out there. I don't know if I should be impressed or appalled. Mostly, I think it's funny. It must be nice.

My mom is not an easy person to summarize. She is not perfect. None of us are. But when things got hard, she showed up. I can attest to that because I was there for some of the hardest things a person can face, and I watched her show up every single time.

Including the summer in Florida when two of her children almost died.

* * *

By then my mom had remarried. His name was Bruce.

He was single and had custody of his three children when they met. He and my mom had met at a local tavern called the Fall Inn in Rose City, Michigan, through a friend. From what I hear it was not love at first sight. She couldn't stand him at first, but he grew on her after a while. He was short and stocky with brownish-red curly hair, a reddish beard, and he always sported a beer belly. One of my first memories of him is from that bar.

My mom would order Sal and me Shirley Temples, and we would play Pac-Man while the adults adulted. I have this perfect memory of him sitting on the barstool with his arms folded over as he did. The red in his beard was really showing that night, and his face was a little shiny. He looked down at me with the biggest smile, the warmest heart. His eyes even had a little glisten about them. Bruce gave Sal the nickname Sally Zuki that afternoon. He was a complicated man. But that is where I want to start with him. At the barstool. With that glisten in his eyes.

* * *

That summer we were in Florida staying at my grandparents while our house in Edgewood was being built. I was eight years old.

I woke up in the camp trailer, and I just did not feel right. My head was pounding to the beat of my heart. My body ached. My eyes could barely open because the light sent a piercing pain straight through my head. I sat up, looked over at Sal, who was still sleeping, and wiped some sweat from my forehead. I waited for my eyes to focus and my head to quit pounding. It didn't. I bent over to grab my shoes, and when I stood back up, I felt dizzy and had to grab the wall to steady myself. I wanted to throw up.

When I walked into my grandparents' house, my mom glanced over at me, looked away, and then her head snapped back towards me. She reached for me and pulled me close. I had red spots from head to toe, and I was burning up with a fever.

She ran a cold bath with baking soda in it. As they thought I might have the measles.

I put one foot in and felt an instant jolt run through my body. I did not want to put the other foot in, but my mother was holding my arm and guiding me in. I stood there shivering stiffly. I sat down with a splash and my teeth chattering, and I felt goose bumps cover my entire body. My head was spinning, and I could barely keep my eyes open. Everything was blurry and too bright. After what felt like an hour but was probably ten minutes, my mom helped me out, and I just leaned into her, shaking and crying.

My mom swears to this day that the water wasn't that cold. I beg to differ. Or maybe that is just what happens when you have a temperature of 103 degrees.

The next morning, my little brother Sal woke up looking just like me.

My mom spent that day on the phone trying to find a doctor's office that would see us. We didn't have insurance, and that was a huge problem. She finally got an appointment at a clinic in town. We were carried to the car. Both of us were whining that the light was too bright and it was too cold. When we got to the doctor's office, a woman came out and rushed us back. She had gloves and a mask on. She looked like one of the characters from E.T.

I was so weak that I just laid right down on the floor. I didn't care that my nightgown, or maybe it was a shirt that had rolled up and was only covering half my body, was clinging tightly around my chest. My mom was only five foot two, heavily pregnant with her third child, and she was trying to carry us both by herself.

A nurse helped me onto the table, where I quickly flopped down. I just wanted to sleep. She then pulled down my panties and took my temperature rectally. Mind you, I was eight years old. That should have bothered me. It did not. I did not care in the least. I was too sick to care about anything.

"103.2," she said.

Next was Sal.

"102.5," the nurse announced.

They gave us suppositories to help bring down the fever and sent us home. One doctor out of all the ones she had called told her that if we got worse, to bring us to the ER, and he would meet us there.

Two days later, we were worse than ever.

Within days, my mom got a hold of the doctor, who said to call him if we didn't get any better, and he sent us to the ER. Once we arrived and after many attempts, they got my IV in. Sal was next. Our room seemed large and had two beds. Sal's was closest to the door, and mine was by the window. Soon after getting settled, they came in for the spinal tap. They had me scrunch up in a ball and told me to sit still. The nurse kept telling me how good I was doing and how brave I was. The poke was deep, but I did not move. Then it was Sal's turn. They told him to pretend he was a wrestler and squeeze his knees to his chest. The nurse wrapped herself around him to make sure he didn't move. They poked him, and he let out a squeal. They kept telling him what a big boy he was, and then it was over.

Days later, Bruce came to see us. He was furious.

"What did you get into?" he demanded. "What did you touch? What did you eat?"

His face was red. His eyebrows were furrowed the way I had seen before when we were in trouble, except this time he seemed more agitated than I had ever seen him. He was pacing the floor.

"We didn't touch anything," we said. "We didn't eat anything. We don't know what happened."

The you're-a-lying-little-shit look was very prominent on his face. He kept ranting. He kept pacing. These were the actions of a scared man.

Once he left, my mom reassured us that he had only been behaving that way because he loved us and didn't want anything bad to happen to us. That she believed us. But if we had done something, it was okay to tell her. We repeated it again. We didn't do anything.

That night, Sal had a nightmare. He was sitting straight up in bed with his arms flailing, tubes, and blood pressure cuff and all, yelling, "I'm gonna give these to Jennifer!" As I looked over half asleep, I saw my mom trying to contain his arms and keep him from pulling out the IV while not startling him fully awake. Sal had always been a sleepwalker. Once back in Michigan, he walked into the living room and was standing in the corner, bumping into the wall. When they asked what he was doing, he said he was going to the bathroom. That was stopped just in time.

As the days went by, we endured more pricking, more poking, more vomiting, more pounding headaches. I couldn't even walk to the bathroom anymore. I was so weak. I remember a young male nurse scooping me up and carrying me to the bathroom because the bedpan had been too hard for me to lift myself onto. When he brought me back to bed, the phone in our room rang, and my mom answered it. I heard her say, "Oh no. How much is that going to cost? At least he is okay." She hung up and shook her head. Our dog had just been bitten between the eyes by a snake. A big fat bill later, Carisa was fine, but still. She looked over at us and said, "What's next?"

That might be something we should never ask the universe. Trust me, it never ends well.

Days later, they still had no clue what was wrong with us. Sal and I were sleeping the day away, losing control of our bowels, and the doctors had run out of explanations. They told my mom it was time to call the family in.

So, she made the calls. She called my dad. Then she called Bruce to tell him they were recommending bringing in the family. He was shocked and told her he had gotten poison oak and was itchy and burning to no end. She sat there shaking her head. “Just look at what kind of luck I have,” she said.

At some point, my grandmother came back to the hospital. This time, she had a magazine article in her hand.

The article was about a case of Rocky Mountain Spotted Fever. The symptoms listed were: high temperature, red spots, lethargy, and sensitivity to light. The list went on. The symptoms were a match.

She showed it to my doctor, and since the blood test would take weeks to come back, they started treating us for it, hoping that was what was wrong with us. They had nothing to lose at that point.

What we learned later was that by then, the doctors had given me one day to live. Sal had two. Grandma walked in just in time.

A couple of days later, I opened my eyes, and my mom looked more distressed than I had ever seen her. She was on the verge of tears, and she looked more tired than I had ever seen another person look. She said quietly, "I am going to go have the baby now. I don't know if they will let me come back in to see you guys because they still don't know if you're contagious or not."

I hugged her, and I cried. She walked over and hugged Sal as well. Then she headed out the door.

She gave birth to a cute six-pound brown-eyed little boy, whom they named Blayne. To only later be nicknamed the cool-aid kid by his favorite sister. Me, of course. He was a cute kid. With a big smile. It fit. Plus, I had caught him with that red ring from it a time or two.

Can you imagine being my poor mom in that situation? Two children extremely ill in the hospital, nobody had any answers. Who do you sit with? Whose hand do you hold? Plus, she had to leave them to give birth. I did not think about any of that at the time. I was eight years old, and I just cried when she walked out the door. I think about it now, though.

Within days of the treatment, Sal was feeling better. He was able to sit up. He was even able to play with some toys.

However, I was still not allowed out of bed. Oddly, I didn't even care that much. I was more concerned about whether Sal would find his way back to the room. I sat there looking at the tube in my arm with blood flowing back up into it, wondering if they would need to change it again. As I watched TV, I faded in and out.

The day before we were released, my dad showed up. I hadn't seen him in a while. He was never good at showing up when he said he would back then. Back home, we had stood by our living room window more than once, looking out at the road, waiting for a car that never came. Getting excited every time headlights approached, only to watch them speed on past.

He showed up this time, and he brought a woman with him. Apparently, he had gotten married. Her name was Loni. She had three kids of her own and they would go on to have two more together. She had her hair dyed blond and she wore blue eyeshadow. Just like my mom. She seemed nice enough. But there was just too much history in that room. Everyone behaved. But you could feel it.

When it was time to leave the hospital, my dad asked if we wanted to ride to my grandma's with him, but my mom would only let one of us go, and since Sal was shy, I knew he would do better with my mom. So, I rode with my dad. He pulled up in a T-Bird with T-tops. The back seat smelled like smoke, and his driving made me want to puke. I tried to make small talk, but my brain felt off. Heavy. Like it was running through water.

When we got to my grandparents he and Loni stayed for a brief moment. He hugged us, said he was so happy we were out of the hospital and was so happy to see us, said "I love you," and then he was gone.

While we were in the hospital, the property in Edgewood, the one we were supposed to be moving to, burned down. We came home from nearly dying to wondering if the house would be okay. My mom never made it sound like a big deal at the time. I don't know if that was for our sake or because, by then, she simply didn't have anything left to spend being upset about it.

We did not get many visitors. My grandmother came often and Bruce came once. That was it outside of my mom. Grandma came even though she had just lost her job and had every reason in the world to be consumed by her own problems. She came anyway. She sat down. She dealt the cards.

We played Gin Rummy and Crazy Eights as I got better. I don't know how many hands we played. Time in a hospital when you are very sick does not move the way time usually moves. What I remember is her sitting there. Steady. Showing up.

I remember my brother during that time, too. Sal was six years old. He had big, chocolate brown eyes and two cowlicks right in the front of his head that stuck straight up no matter what anyone did with them. We called them his little devil horns. He was, by all accounts, an extraordinarily cute little boy, and the nurses absolutely adored him.

When a nurse would come in and needed Sal to do something, and if we were alone, he would look at me first. Just a glance. His big brown eyes finding mine across the room. Checking in. Making sure it was okay. And when I was aware enough to catch it, I would give him a nod. Yep. Listen to the lady. And he would.

We were so young, and my little brother was looking to me for confirmation that the world was safe. I did not think about that at the time, but writing this made me think about it now.

We watched a lot of TV too, if you want to call it that. What I actually did was watch for about three minutes, feel my eyelids getting heavy, sleep for an hour, wake up, watch for another three minutes, and repeat. The TV was more of a background presence than something I actually watched. I was too sick to follow anything for long. But the sound of it was comforting. Something ordinary in a place that felt anything but.

Grandma loved to bake, to thrift, and to fish. We went fishing together often when I got a little older. We hit garage sales on weekends, and she taught me that the best things in life were the ones you found for almost nothing. I still believe that. I still do all of those things. When I find something good at a garage sale, I think of her.

She remarried when I was young. My grandpa, Ken, had a strong southern accent and ran his own business fixing washers and dryers. When I got older, he would take me with him sometimes on service calls. We went to some pretty fancy houses. He also sang in a band at night in bars. My grandmother would go and watch and cheer him on; she was his biggest fan. I remember dancing the night away in a South Prairie Tavern. Kids were allowed in bars back then and I never thought twice about being in one. Kids in bars were a common occurrence back then.

Grandma, my mom, and I also volunteered together at the Orting Eagles during the Daffodil Parade, where I handed out hot dogs. It was a small thing, but it meant something to me, being part of the community, watching people come together, doing something useful, even if it was an itty-bitty part. That was Grandma, too. She found ways to show up for people. Big and small.

Anyway, once we got home from the hospital, my body did not get that memo.

I was tired in a way I had never been tired before. Not sleepy tired. Heavy tired. Like something was sitting on top of my head pressing down, and no matter how much I slept, it was still there when I woke up. I went back to school and sat at my desk trying to learn cursive and multiplication, and the words and numbers on the page would blur, and my chin would drop toward my chest, and I would be out. Just like that. I never got comfortable with multiplication after that. To this day, I do my nines on my fingers. You know the trick, you put all ten fingers up, put down the first one, and that's one times nine. Put it back up and put down the second finger, and that's two times nine, eighteen. It's a magical trick that has kept me in nine's purgatory my whole life.

My iron levels were dangerously low. My mom was told that I needed iron and protein, and she took that seriously in the way only a certain kind of mother can, the kind who does not negotiate and does not apologize.

She made liver.

I want to be fair and tell you I tried. I really did. I put it in my mouth, and the texture hit my tongue, and something primal in me recoiled. It tasted like a key and it left a sticky, velvety film in my mouth that no amount of water would wash away. There was gagging. Then, there was a brief and unsuccessful attempt to swallow it whole without chewing. Then there was more gagging.

My mom stood firm.

It was Halloween, and my brother and I had been looking forward to it more than we ever had before. After being in the hospital for two weeks, something as simple as candy, costumes, and being outside felt like the most normal and wonderful thing in the world.

We were not going, she informed us, until we ate the liver.

I will not tell you how that night ended because I honestly don't remember if we made it out the door. What I remember is that it was a very long night and that I still hate liver with every fiber of my being and no amount of iron deficiency will ever change that.

Some battles cannot be won.

The liver battle was one of them, but that wasn't the only thing that year had in store for me.

They held me back. Third grade. Same grade. Again.

I had fallen too far behind. Falling asleep at my desk hadn't helped. Nobody pulled me aside and explained it in a way that made sense. Nobody said your body went through something serious, and it takes time, and that is okay.

Everyone else moved forward. I stayed.

I don't say that to be dramatic. I say it because nobody talks about what comes after surviving something like this. The doctors did their job. They saved our lives. But they sent us home, and the rest of it, the heaviness and the falling asleep and the year that looked different from everyone else's. That was just ours to figure out. To be fair, I don't think anyone knew what we were going through. It wasn't like they sent us home saying there could be a recovery period or anything.

I figured it out. Kids do.

As it turned out, I didn't have to face my friends at recess either. We changed schools before the next school year began. So, it was like it never happened. Almost.

As I got better, I remember watching Spaceballs. Mel Brooks' Star Wars parody, which came out in 1987. By then, I was home and recovering and capable of watching something for more than three minutes without falling asleep, which felt like an achievement. I remember laughing at it. I remember that laughing felt good. That is what I remember about getting better more than anything else. The return of the ability to laugh at something ridiculous for an hour and a half.

* * *

Life in the mid-eighties had a specific texture that I don't think any other era has quite replicated. Everything was bright and I mean that literally. The colors were loud and unapologetic. Neon everything. Hot pink and electric blue, and a particular shade of orange and yellow that had no business being on a piece of clothing but was absolutely everywhere. If the seventies were earthy and the nineties were grunge, the eighties were a decade that had decided subtlety was for other cool people.

And cartoons. I cannot talk about this period of my life without talking about the cartoons.

He-Man and the Masters of the Universe had taken over everything. He-Man was the most powerful man in the universe, which he announced out loud every single episode while holding a sword above his head and transforming from Prince Adam into something considerably more impressive. The premise was gloriously simple. Good versus evil. He-Man versus Skeletor. Castle Grayskull was at stake every week, and somehow it was always saved. The animation was not particularly smooth, and it had a moral lessons at the end of each episode. We were obsessed.

Then there was She-Ra, she was He-Man's twin sister, she had her own show and her own sword and castle, and she was, if anything, even more powerful and considerably more fabulous. She-Ra: Princess of Power premiered in 1985 and immediately became part of the fabric of being a girl in the mid-eighties. She had friends.

She had allies. She had an army. She was kind and fierce in equal measure, and she did not wait around to be rescued. In a decade that was just beginning to figure out what female heroes could look like on screen, She-Ra was a significant thing during that time. Hell, I think she may need to make a come back today! Little girls could really use a role model like her.

And then there were the ThunderCats.

Lion-O. Cheetara. Tygra. Panthro. A group of humanoid cat warriors from a dying planet crash-land on a new world and fighting evil with a magical sword called the Sword of Omens. The catchphrase was Thunder, Thunder, ThunderCats, HO, delivered at maximum volume by a boy king holding a glowing sword toward the sky. I loved them without apology. You could hear us and the neighbor kids screaming, "THUNDER CATS HOOOO" with our harms raised in the air. Pretending to hold up our swords.

These were the things filling up the hours of being a kid in 1985 and 1986. Bright colors. Big heroes. Clear lines between good and evil. A world that felt, at least on television, like it made a certain amount of sense.

And then on a cold January morning in 1986, a Tuesday, everything stopped making sense for a while.

* * *

There had been enormous excitement in the lead-up to the Challenger launch. The reason was Christa McAuliffe, a high school social studies teacher from New Hampshire who had been selected through NASA's Teacher in Space program to become the first civilian to fly on the space shuttle. The idea was to bring space closer to everyday Americans. To make it feel possible and real and connected to ordinary life. Schools across the country were invited to watch the launch live. Teachers gathered their students. We stood in single-file lines and went outside.

I remember standing there in the Florida cold. January 28, 1986, was unusually cold for Florida. There had been ice on the launch pad. We didn't know that then. We were just kids standing in a line watching the sky.

The shuttle launched. You could see it. A bright streak climbing upward, leaving its trail against the blue.

And then, seventy-three seconds after liftoff, it was gone.

Not gone the way something disappears over the horizon. Gone the way something breaks apart. A plume of smoke and debris where a moment before there had been a spacecraft. The plume split into two trails curving away from each other like arms opening wide, and then there was nothing where the shuttle had been.

The gasp that went through our group was something I have never forgotten. It was not individual gasps. It was one sound from all of us at once, involuntary, and immediate, the sound a crowd makes when it witnesses something it cannot immediately process. And then the crying started. Kids around me crying. Teachers moving us back inside with an urgency that had nothing to do with the cold.

I don't remember what was said inside the classroom after that. I don't remember a conversation. I don't remember a counselor coming to talk to us. In 1986, the idea of bringing in grief counselors for children who had witnessed a national tragedy was not standard practice, the way it is now. We went back inside. We probably went back to our lessons at some point. Life moved on the way life moves on.

Seven people died on the Challenger. Christa McAuliffe, the teacher, was one of them. She had wanted to bring space to the classroom. She brought something else instead, something that stayed with me for a long time. The understanding that even things built by brilliant people with the best intentions and the highest stakes can go catastrophically wrong in a moment.

I was eight years old, and I had already almost died twice. I understood something about that already.

And to this day, I always question what I saw that day. Was I really standing outside watching it in the sky, or were we watching it on the little TV on the big grey stand with wheels on it, that got rolled into classrooms for special occasions? I honestly cannot say for certain. What I do know is that I saw it. What I felt standing there or sitting there was real. The gasp was real. The crying was real. Memory does funny things to the details, but it never forgets the feeling.

* * *

Things were getting back to normal. The scars from when the Doberman attacked me had left a mark in several places: my neck, my shoulder, my upper arm, and the back of my right leg. Luckily, they are small, but deep enough to leave their mark. The kind of scars that become part of your geography, things you stop noticing after a while because they have always just been there. Just like the cigarette scar on my left cheek. I earned that bad boy by standing up in the back seat of the car, playing with my brother, when my dad had to slam on the brakes. He had put his arm back, with his cigarette in hand, to stop me from going out of the windshield, and he accidentally put his cigarette out on my face. The scar normally doesn't bother me, but these days it's changing color. Looking for attention. Being all dramatic and shit.

You would think that would have taught me not to play around in the backseat, but when I was six or so, we were playing in the backseat of my mom's car, and a police officer used his loudspeaker to tell us to sit down. I have never heard a police officer use his loudspeaker since. Nowadays, I think you would just get a big fat ticket. Oh, the good old eighties.

* * *

Those scars healed. They faded. They became a part of me. Until one morning, when the deepest one, the one on my neck felt different. It was itchy. I reached back and felt around, and there was something there. Something that shouldn't be.

I went inside and found my mom and grandmother sitting in the kitchen smoking their cigarettes and chatting as they did. My mom started putting my hair up in a ponytail the way she always did, and I told her I felt something in my scar.

She went quiet for a second.

Then she saw it.

"You have got to be fucking kidding me."

She caught herself immediately.

"Oh no. Don't freak out. It's okay." A pause. "Ugh, I hate these damn things."

My grandmother came over to look. They exchanged a glance over my head that I absolutely clocked and pretended I hadn't.

"Sit still," my mom said.

She got the tweezers.

I sat there and let her work it out of the deepest part of my scar, and I did not move. Tears were welling up, and I was grossed out in a way that went through my bones, but I held still. I had learned how to hold still. I had learned it the hard way, in that hospital bed, with a needle in my spine while someone told me I was brave.

Of all the places. A tick had found the one spot on my body that was already scarred. Already damaged. And made itself right at home there.

I was grossed out for weeks afterward.

Honestly, I still am, just thinking about it right now.

* * *

A few months after we got out of the hospital, I had an extra molar growing in alongside my regular teeth and the dentist said it needed to come out. A simple, routine procedure. When they got the needle ready to numb my mouth, I looked at it and felt heat run throughout my body, and my heart start racing. Then, with a burst of energy, I stood up and ripped the tooth out myself. I think I shocked myself as much as anyone else in that room.

The dental assistant stared at me. Her mouth opened, and nothing came out.

My mom's eyes went wide. "What the hell," she said.

The dental assistant then said, "Ok, let me take a look." Wiped my lip and said, "I guess we are done here" and we headed out.

Then later, once the shock wore off, my mom looked at me and said, "Well, if you could just pull it out, why didn't you do that at home?" We laughed.

We still got billed for that visit. My mom was appalled. I agreed wholeheartedly. I mean, I did all the work.

What the hospital gave me, along with my life, was a very specific relationship with my own body. A knowledge that I could handle more than people expected. A low tolerance for waiting around while someone else decided what was going to happen to me.

I am not recommending anyone pull their own tooth out.

But I understand, in my bones, why I did it.

And I think if you had been in that hospital bed, you might understand it too.

Chapter 3:

Five Whats???

Our daughter Hailey was going to Eastern Washington University, and we drove out to Spokane to visit her for the weekend.

It was a beautiful day. The kind of day that makes you forget to worry about anything. Hailey suggested we check out Turnbull National Wildlife Refuge, a walking path nearby that she had heard about. It sounded perfect. So, we headed out after lunch.

On the way there, we spotted a moose.

"MOOSE!" Hailey yelled from the back seat. "I think I saw a moose!" John said it almost at the same time. "A moose." He glanced in the rear-view mirror, confirmed the road was empty behind us, and put the car in reverse. We crept back slowly. And there she was. John looked at her and said it quietly. “Yep. There’s Rebekah.” Hailey and I looked at each other. “Rebekah? What?” We all laughed. Before we headed home, we went looking for her one more time. No Rebekah. Gone just like that.

We have been hunting for moose for years. We once made a trip to Yellowstone, and stayed at a campsite specifically known for sightings, and came home without seeing a single one. Then on the drive back through Washington, we spotted one standing in a marsh off the side of the road. The first moose any of us had ever seen. Just standing there. Like she had been waiting for us. Almost as if she was mocking us even. You silly humans drove all that way, and I have just been hanging out here this whole time.

After lunch, Hailey had things to do, so John and I headed to the refuge on our own.

We were in good spirits when we got to the refuge. The path was paved for the most part, with long grass here and there crossing over it in places. Nothing dramatic. Nothing that screamed danger. It was one of the last summer days of the year, and we were just walking and talking and enjoying being together. We were alone for the most part. Afterward, we also walked through a civil war reenactment happening nearby. People were dressed for the time, with the long draping dresses, and the men looking so dapper in their uniforms, guns in tow. Here, the grass was longer, and we moved through it without thinking much of it. It was all just part of the day.

* * *

That evening, we were getting ready to go swimming at the hotel and John had taken off his shirt, and I noticed what looked like speckled moles on his back.

I moved closer, and my stomach dropped.

They weren't moles.

They were ticks. Multiple ticks. Embedded in my husband's back like they had been there for hours, which, as it turns out, they probably had.

I got the creepy crawlies immediately. The full body kind. The kind that starts at the back of your neck, works its way down to your feet, and makes your skin feel like it belongs to someone else. Or you wish that it did.

I am not a fan of ticks. But I pulled it together. I hesitantly sterilized the tweezers. I mean, he couldn't exactly reach his own back and it was just John and me.

I got as close to the skin as I could and removed them one by one. Slowly. Carefully. Trying not to think too hard about what I was doing while also thinking about nothing else.

If you were to ask John about it today, he would say there were only three tick. However, I say there were five. I was the one doing the removing, so I would think my count is more reliable. But we will never fully agree on that number, and at this point, it has become its own running joke.

Growing up, I had seen ticks removed from animals with a lit lighter, touching the flame close enough to make them back out on their own. It was just what people did. My family did it. A lot of families did. But the recommended method now is to avoid that entirely. Heat can actually cause a tick to release more saliva or stomach contents into the wound, which is the last thing you want. The right way is straight upward pressure with fine-tipped tweezers, as close to the skin as possible, without twisting or jerking. Clean the bite area afterward with rubbing alcohol or soap and water. Then you can add an antibiotic type ointment like bacitracin.

That is what I did. One by one. Slow and steady.

When it was over, I disposed of them, and we went swimming and tried to move on with our evening.

* * *

Except I couldn't move on.

Almost immediately after I threw them away, I thought, wait. Should I have kept those?

The answer, as I would learn that night, was yes. I mean, I did know it, but my mind was also telling me, we don't have dangerous ticks in Washington. Do we? I just couldn't recall or maybe that's just what I wanted to believe

I spent the rest of the evening on my phone looking up tick species in Washington, what to watch for after a bite, whether the type of tick mattered for the kind of illness you could get, and how long you had to have been bitten before transmission was possible. I needed a refresher. It had been a while since I had thought much about these little monsters. I don't remember exactly what I found, but I remember that it made me look harder. It made me pay attention again. It sparked my curiosity about ticks and how such a tiny thing can be so harmful to us big humans.

I watched John for days, and nothing developed. We were lucky.

But I have thought about that evening more than once since then. Because here is the thing, we were on a paved path. It was a beautiful sunny day. We were not bushwhacking through wilderness or camping in tall grass. We were just walking. And John came home with five ticks on his back.

It doesn't take much. That is the part people don't fully understand until it happens to them. You don't have to be doing anything dramatic. You just have to be outside.

* * *

If I could go back, I would have saved those ticks in a small, sealed plastic bag.

I regretted throwing them away almost immediately. That instinct was right, too.

So, if you find one, save it. A sealed zip-lock bag in the freezer works fine. Write the date on it. Note where you were when you found it. It costs you nothing, and it could matter more than you know.

Oh, and check yourself and your family after every walk. Even the paved ones.

We named a moose Rebekah that day. We also got a good reminder of just how quickly and easily a tick can enter your life.

Chapter 4:

It Was Always Going to Be Me

I want to be honest about something before I tell you this part of the story.

I am not some kind of superhuman observer. I did not notice everything. I did not catch every warning sign. When my oldest son was a teen, he was sneaking out and doing drugs, and I had no idea. Not a clue. I found out the way most parents find out, which is later than you want to and not in a way that feels good. Although, it did lead us to discover that he had a lesion on his brain.

My oldest was a stubborn child. He was not one to take responsibility. And while that was happening, the chaos he was creating at home had a way of spreading. My second son and my daughter got caught in the crossfire more than once, taking heat for things that weren't theirs to carry.

I tell you this because I want you to understand what I mean when I say I am not exceptional. I was paying close attention to the wrong things while something significant was happening under my own roof. That was humbling. It still is.

My oldest is doing well now. He is a dad and a husband. My second son works at a hospital and is also doing well in life. I am proud of both of them. But I want to be honest about the fact that the same person who pushed for answers in doctors' offices and hospital waiting rooms missed what was happening in her own house. Paying attention is not a superpower. It is practice. And some days you practice it better than others.

So, when I tell you that I have a knack for knowing when something is medically wrong with the people I love, I am not telling you that I am exceptional. I am telling you that life gave me a lot of practice.

My husband John and I have been together for twenty-five years. He is the kind of man who does not complain, does not worry out loud, and does not go to the doctor unless someone makes him. That someone has always been me. I don't say that to take credit for anything. I say it because by the time something started shifting with John, I had spent decades learning how to read the people I love.

The first thing I noticed was the hair.

John was a hairy man. Everywhere but his head, as he would tell you himself. But one day, I noticed the hair on his body was disappearing. Not gradually, the way these things sometimes go. Just… gone. Then he started hitting the snooze button. This was a man who had never in our years together needed an alarm to get him out of bed. He was a get-up-and-go kind of person who was suddenly struggling to get up at all. Then the mobility issues started. Small things at first. Things you could explain away if you wanted to.

I didn't.

It took me two years to convince him to get a physical. John is a stubborn man, and we were coming off the back of COVID when everything medical felt complicated and overwhelming, and like one more thing nobody wanted to deal with. He kept putting it off. I kept pushing.

I was so worried that at a certain point, I quietly bought term life insurance. I didn't make a big announcement about it. I just did it. Because I knew something was wrong and I was trying to be practical about what that might mean, while still refusing to stop fighting for an answer. That is the space you live in when you love someone who won't take care of themselves. Hope in one hand. Contingency plan in the other.

I had been paying $350 a month, and I am still paying it today. We have our answer now. He has been through brain surgery, and he is still here. That is the most relieved I have ever been to still be writing that check. Even at that price.

* * *

Then, there was my dad, he called it random chest pain. Pressure, he said. Some achiness. Occasional shortness of breath but nothing serious. He was not planning to go to the doctor.

My stepmom mentioned it to me one day when I was visiting. We were sitting at their kitchen table while she smoked a cigarette and drank her beer, the way you mention something when you are hoping someone else will take it seriously, so you don't have to be the one to push.

I looked at my dad. He seemed clammy. Pale. Off in a way that was hard to name but impossible to ignore once you saw it. As he heard us talking about him. He then said, "I just have a little tingling and numbness in my arm. It feels weird."

That was it. I knew.

I did not gently suggest he see a doctor. I got rude. I told him he could die. I told him it did not matter if he didn't have insurance or if there were going to be bills. I told him his life was more important than any of that and that we were going. Then, I told him to stop being selfish and get ready to go.

He went.

They put in two stents. I was in the room during the procedure, watching him in a twilight state, listening to him tell them when he felt discomfort as they worked. Afterward, when it was over, and he was coming back to himself, he looked at me and said it quietly.

"I guess it's a good thing you made me come."

My dad's story took one afternoon and ended with seven words. John's took two years. And before both of them, there was Blayne.

He called me and told me that he had a horrible headache, his eyes hurt, he had a fever, and his neck felt stiff. I asked him if he had been outside a lot. I thought maybe it was heat stroke and he said that he had. So, I told him that if it got worse, to go to the ER. The next thing I know, my mom called me and said Blayne went to the ER. Apparently, she had also told him to go. By the time my mom got there, he was on a gurney, and the evaluation had begun. There was one nurse who took one look at him and indicated immediately that she knew what he had and that they needed to act fast. They discussed putting him into a medical coma so they could control the swelling in his brain. It was all very tricky. Blayne was considered an adult, being nineteen, so making decisions was complicated. All medical decisions were made by the doctors until he woke up and signed paperwork allowing my mom to speak for him, but by then, there weren't really any decisions to be made.

The first couple of nights, we stayed vigil overnight at the hospital. On about day three, the power went out. My mom and I had been walking out of his room toward the elevator when everything went dark. My instinct was to run back to the room, and that is exactly what my body did. My mom quickly grabbed my arm and said, "What are you going to do, breathe for him?" And just then, the backup generator kicked on. We still went and checked on him. Then we went outside to smoke. And then we laughed. I don't know what I thought I was going to do but it was something.

They had him on a ventilator. You could hear the sound of the machine as it took breaths for him. The bed was maroon and it had sheets on it, but you could still see it. It was a rotating bed. I had never seen one before. His upper right side would go up, and his lower left side would go down. It was like the bed was moving to the sound of some unknown melody. It was scary to see the deep purple spots appearing on his hands and legs. Up to his knees. At that point, everything was still unknown.

He came home almost two weeks later. He had wounds that needed care for a long time after. He got lucky and is fully functional today. He only carries his survivor scars. Badges of honor, really. He beat a very deadly illness.

I think about my mother sometimes and what she has carried in her lifetime. All three of her children. Two different life-threatening illnesses. Sal and I nearly died from Rocky Mountain Spotted Fever in that Florida hospital when I was eight and Sal was around six years old. Then, years later, her son Blayne was in the ICU in a medical coma. Three children. Two separate times, she was told she might lose one of us.

I don't know what you call that kind of luck. I just know that if there was ever a woman who earned the right to fall apart, she was standing right there. And she never did. She is the ultimate shit streak survivor.

What Blayne had was meningococcal meningitis, caused by the bacterium Neisseria meningitidis. It is rare, and it moves fast. According to the CDC, in 2024, there were 503 confirmed and probable cases reported nationwide. The highest number in the United States since before 2014 and rising. With a population of over 330 million people, your odds in a normal year are roughly less than one in 100,000 for the average healthy adult. But those odds mean nothing when it is your family member on the ventilator.

The disease spreads through close contact, coughing, kissing, living with someone, and sharing drinks. It is not spread through casual contact or by breathing air in a room where someone infected has been. Young adults living in close quarters, college dormitories, and military barracks, are at higher risk. People with HIV are disproportionately affected in the current rise in cases.

Symptoms come on fast and can look like something else at first. Fever. Severe headache. Stiff neck. Nausea and vomiting. Sensitivity to light. Confusion or altered mental status. In later stages, a dark purple rash can appear on the hands and legs. Blayne had those marks. I saw them with my own eyes. The disease can become life-threatening within hours. Immediate antibiotic treatment is critical.

There are vaccines. The CDC recommends MenACWY for all preteens and teens and for adults at increased risk. If you have a child heading to college, ask about meningococcal vaccination.

* * *

By the time John's changes became impossible to ignore, I had already sat vigil through my stepdad's five-way bypass and kidney transplant. I had been there for my mom through her ear surgery, jaw surgery, neck surgery, and bladder surgery. I had advocated for Blayne when I felt I should and I helped with wound care after he came home too. I had forced my dad to go to the hospital when he was about to have a heart attack and didn't want to go. A total close call.

Some of those situations I fought for. Others I simply showed up for. Both matter. But the fighting ones taught me something the showing up ones couldn't, which is that the difference between a good outcome and a bad one is often the one person who speaks up.

What I have learned, through all of it, is that bodies tell the truth even when people don't. You just have to know how to listen.

I share this because it illustrates something I want you to understand. The person who saves someone is very rarely the most educated person in the room. Sometimes, like with Blayne, the educated person catches it fast and that is its own kind of luck. But more often, it is the person paying the closest attention and willing to speak up even when they are afraid of being wrong. I was afraid of being wrong too. I am always afraid of being wrong. I speak up anyway.

I did not think about any of this consciously when things started changing with John. I did not sit down and say to myself. I have a history of catching things other people miss; let me apply that skill here.

It was not like that. It was instinct. Something was wrong, and I knew it, the way you know something is wrong before you can explain why. The way my grandmother knew when she read that magazine article. Not because she had been trained to look for it. Because she was paying attention, and something matched.

John was tired in a way that sleep wasn't fixing. The hair on his body was disappearing. The man who had never been able to keep his hands off me had gone quiet in a way that had nothing to do with us. And when they finally tested his testosterone at my request. It came back at a level of 3. I was surprised. I thought it was the issue, but I did not expect a number so low.

I wrote the notes before every appointment. I pushed for every test. I couldn't find anything about a level of 3 anywhere and that had me stunned and worried.

Eventually, we found a pituitary tumor the size of a grape wrapped around his internal carotid artery and had brain surgery.

Although, before they even told us about his tumor I had figured it out. I wasn't one hundred percent sure, but I was pretty sure. I thought about my grandmother that day after I found out that I was right about Johns diagnosis.

She did not have medical training. She was not a doctor. She was a woman who picked up a magazine, paid attention, and refused to brush it off.

I did not have medical training either. I was just someone who had spent a lifetime watching people she loved and learning that bodies tell the truth if you listen closely enough.

I am not telling you this to take credit for saving my husband's life. I am telling you this because the through line matters.

My grandmother passed something to me in that Florida hospital room, whether she meant to or not. Not a lesson. Not advice. Just a way of being in the world. Present. Attentive. Willing to speak up.

I have tried to pass the same thing to the people around me.

Including you.

It might be nothing. But if it's something, you'll be glad you didn't stay quiet.

Pay attention. Trust what you see.

Don't brush it off.

Rocky Mountain Spotted Fever: What You Need to Know

You have already read what this disease did to my brother and me in 1985. Now let me tell you what it actually is, why it is so dangerous, and why it keeps catching people off guard even today.

Because it is still out there, and it is still being missed forty years later.

* * *

What Is It?

Rocky Mountain Spotted Fever is a bacterial disease caused by Rickettsia rickettsii, a type of bacteria carried primarily by three tick species: the American dog tick, the Rocky Mountain wood tick, and the brown dog tick. Despite the name, it is found throughout the United States and into Central and South America nowadays. It is not limited to mountains. It is not limited to the West. It can happen anywhere those ticks live, which is nearly everywhere.

In the United States, the highest concentration of cases is actually in the south and southeast, particularly in North Carolina, Oklahoma, Arkansas, Tennessee, and Missouri. Cases have been documented in all 48 contiguous states.

My brother and I got it in Florida. From ticks nobody ever found.

* * *

Why It Is So Dangerous

RMSF attacks the walls of your blood vessels. Once the bacteria enter your bloodstream, they begin damaging the lining of vessels throughout your entire body, which can lead to organ failure, neurological damage, and death. This is why it progresses so rapidly and why delays in treatment are so deadly.

Without treatment, death can occur within eight days of symptoms starting. That is not a typo. Eight days. A healthy person with no prior conditions can go from the first fever to death in eight days if the disease is not caught and treated correctly. Even with treatment, approximately three to five percent of patients will die from it. Without treatment, that number rises to between thirteen and twenty-five percent. Most of those deaths occur when the diagnosis is not made until the second week of illness. With prompt treatment, the survival rate is high. Even among survivors of severe cases, some experience long-term consequences, including hearing loss, partial limb loss, and neurological damage.

My brother and I were given one day and two days, respectively. We were on the edge of that window. My grandmother found the answer just in time.

* * *

The Symptoms

This is where RMSF gets tricky. The early symptoms are almost identical to those of dozens of other illnesses. That is why it gets missed so often.

Early symptoms typically include high fever, often above 102 or 103 degrees; severe headache; body aches and muscle pain; nausea and vomiting; fatigue and general feeling of being unwell; and sensitivity to light.

The rash typically appears two to four days after the fever begins. It usually starts on the wrists and ankles and spreads inward toward the trunk. The spots are small, flat, and pink or red at first. As the disease progresses, they can become darker, more defined, and in severe cases develop into a petechial rash, which involves small bleeding under the skin.

Here is the critical thing most people do not know: not everyone gets the rash. In the early stages, the rash is absent in up to 60 percent of patients. And in some cases, it never fully develops. This means a doctor looking for the classic spotted appearance may not see it, especially in the first few days when treatment would be most effective.

I had red spots head to toe. My brother did too. But that is not always the case. Do not wait for spots to appear before you take action.

* * *

Why It Gets Missed

Several things make RMSF particularly difficult to diagnose.

First, the early symptoms mimic so many other things. Flu. Viral infection. Stomach bug. A doctor seeing a child with high fever, headache, and body aches has dozens of explanations available before they get to tick-borne illness. Especially if there is no visible rash and no known tick bite.

Second, patients often do not know they were bitten. Ticks are small. Their bites are painless. They can attach and feed for hours without you feeling anything. My brother and I had no known tick bites. The doctors checked us when we came in and found no ticks. That alone nearly cost us our lives because it removed tick-borne illness from the differential. Well, that and the fact that two people had never presented at once before.

Third, laboratory tests in the early days are often inconclusive. The blood tests for RMSF are most accurate later in the disease when antibodies have had time to develop. In the first few days when treatment matters most, the tests may come back negative or inconclusive. The CDC recommends that treatment should never be delayed waiting for lab results if RMSF is suspected.

There is also the matter of the name Rocky Mountain Spotted Fever. It sounds like something you would get in the mountains out west. We were in Florida. Cases in Florida were rare in 1985. It is documented but uncommon, and the misleading name meant doctors were not looking for it there. That combination of rarity and a name and two children sick at the same time pointed everyone in the wrong direction, nearly cost us our lives. This is exactly why my grandmother's magazine article mattered. She connected the dots that the hospital could not. She gave them a direction when the tests had given them nothing.

* * *

Treatment

The good news is that RMSF is treatable. The antibiotic doxycycline is the first-line treatment for adults and children of all ages, and it works. The key is starting it quickly.

Treatment is most effective when started within the first five days of symptoms. After that window, the disease can progress faster than the antibiotic can keep up. This is why the recommendation from the CDC is clear: if RMSF is suspected, start treatment immediately. Do not wait for a confirmed diagnosis. Do not wait for the rash. Do not wait for the lab results.

Studies show that patients who begin doxycycline after day five are significantly more likely to die or experience permanent damage than those who start treatment early. Most deaths from RMSF occur in patients who do not receive treatment until the second week of illness. Often, because the diagnosis was missed or delayed.

If you are in an area where ticks are common, if you or your child has been outside recently, and if the symptoms match, tell your doctor you want RMSF considered and treatment started now. Those words could save a life.

Long-Term Effects

What the doctors don't always tell survivors is what can linger. Rocky Mountain Spotted Fever causes vasculitis, which is inflammation and damage to blood vessels throughout the body. That damage can leave marks that don't show up on any discharge paperwork.

Long-term effects in severe cases have included hearing loss, neurological damage, peripheral neuropathy, and, in the worst cases, amputation of fingers, toes, or limbs where blood flow was cut off. A study published in the journal Clinical Infectious Diseases followed 25 patients who had been hospitalized for two or more weeks with severe RMSF. Nearly half still had at least one long-term complication directly related to their original infection. Researchers tracked these patients for up to eighteen years after they were discharged.

Eighteen years.

I fell asleep at my desk for months after I came home. My brain felt like it was running through water. I have had neck and back issues my whole life, which I have always wondered about.

This makes me nervous about my health. I do have heart disease, and I found out young. Related? I will never know. What is more disconcerting is that when I tell doctors I almost died from this as a child, they shrug their shoulders and nod their heads. They never think it has anything to do with it. This is a battle I continue to fight.

I don't know with certainty what is connected and what isn't. However, I do know, I was given one day to live, and I am still here. Whatever I carried out of that hospital, I will take over the alternative every single time.

* * *

The Bottom Line

Rocky Mountain Spotted Fever is one of the most dangerous tick-borne diseases in the United States. It is fast-moving, frequently misdiagnosed, and potentially fatal within days. The rash that gives it its name is often absent in early stages. The tests that confirm it take time, which the patient may not have.

What saves lives is the same thing that saved mine. Someone is paying attention. Someone who sees patterns. Someone who is willing to put themselves out there and speak up.

If you have been outside and you develop a high fever with a severe headache and body aches, especially if you live in or have traveled to an area where ticks are common, tell your doctor. Mention ticks. Ask specifically about RMSF. Ask about doxycycline.

Do not brush it off.

Alpha-Gal Syndrome: The Tick That Steals Red Meat

A 47-year-old man in New Jersey went to a barbecue in September 2024. He ate a hamburger. He died that evening.

The cause was an allergic reaction. Not to the barbecue sauce. Not to anything he had ever been allergic to before. To the beef itself. A reaction triggered not by anything he ate that day, but by a tick bite he may not have even known he received.

He was the first documented death from Alpha-Gal Syndrome in the United States.

He is not the last.

* * *

What Is Alpha-Gal Syndrome?

Alpha-Gal Syndrome, or AGS, is a food allergy to red meat caused by a tick bite. It sounds impossible. It is real.

Here is how it works. Most mammals, including cows, pigs, lambs, and deer, produce a sugar molecule called galactose-alpha-1,3-galactose, or alpha-gal. Humans do not produce this molecule, which means our immune systems can recognize it as foreign.

When a tick bites you, alpha-gal from the tick's saliva enters your bloodstream. In some people, the immune system identifies it as a threat and produces antibodies against it. Once those antibodies exist, eating red meat, which contains alpha-gal, can trigger an allergic reaction. In severe cases, it can trigger anaphylaxis, which is a life-threatening whole-body reaction.

The allergy does not develop in everyone who is bitten. Researchers are still studying why some people become sensitized, and others do not. But the number of people affected is rising dramatically, and the allergy can develop after a single bite you never even noticed.

* * *

The Numbers Are Alarming

According to the CDC, more than 110,000 suspected cases of Alpha-Gal Syndrome were identified in the United States between 2010 and 2022. But because many people with symptoms are never tested, researchers estimate that as many as 450,000 Americans may currently be living with the condition.

That number is growing fast. A study presented at the American College of Gastroenterology's annual meeting in November 2025 analyzed records from more than 3,800 adults tested for alpha-gal antibodies between 2010 and 2025. The findings were striking. Positive test results increased from about 1.8 percent of those tested in 2013 and 2014 to nearly 39 percent in 2021 and 2022. That is a roughly 100-fold increase in about a decade.

Forty-two percent of doctors surveyed by the CDC said they had never heard of Alpha-Gal Syndrome. The condition is spreading faster than awareness of it.

* * *

What Makes It So Hard to Catch

Alpha-Gal Syndrome is unlike almost any other food allergy, and that is exactly what makes it so dangerous and so frequently missed.

Most food allergies cause reactions within minutes. With Alpha-Gal Syndrome, symptoms appear three to six hours after eating. By the time the reaction hits, the meal is a distant memory. A person who eats a burger at six in the evening and wakes up at midnight with hives, stomach pain, or worse has very little reason to connect what is happening to what they ate hours earlier.

This delay happens because the alpha-gal molecule is attached to fats in the meat. The body has to digest and absorb those fats before the molecule enters the bloodstream and triggers the immune response.

Add to that the fact that not every exposure causes the same reaction. Some people have mild symptoms like hives or stomach cramps. Others go into full anaphylaxis. The same person can react differently to different amounts of red meat or at different times.

* * *

Which Tick Causes It?

In the United States, the condition is most commonly associated with the Lone Star tick, which is recognizable by a single white spot on the back of the adult female. The Lone Star tick is found primarily in the eastern and south-central United States, but its range has been expanding northward and westward as temperatures shift.

Some cases have also been reported following bites from blacklegged ticks and western blacklegged ticks. Globally, researchers have identified at least twelve tick species linked to Alpha-Gal Syndrome across every continent except Antarctica.

This is not a regional problem anymore.

* * *

The Bottom Line

If you develop unexplained allergic reactions, particularly in the middle of the night or several hours after meals, especially after eating red meat, tell your doctor and specifically ask about Alpha-Gal Syndrome. Ask for the specific IgE blood test that checks for alpha-gal antibodies. Do not assume your doctor will think of it. Forty-two percent of them have never heard of it.

The man in New Jersey mowed his lawn after eating that hamburger. He felt fine. He had no idea a tick bite had changed everything.

Don't let that be you. Keep watch this tick season.

Lyme Disease: What You Think You Know and What You Don't

Lyme disease is the most talked-about tick-borne illness in America. It is also one of the most misunderstood.

Most people have heard of it. Most people believe they know what it looks like. Many of them are wrong about the most important parts. And those gaps in understanding are exactly why it keeps getting missed.

* * *

What It Is?

Lyme disease is caused by a bacterium called Borrelia burgdorferi, which is spread to humans through the bite of infected blacklegged ticks, also known as deer ticks. It is the most common vector-borne disease in the United States.

According to the CDC, over 89,000 cases of Lyme disease were reported to state health departments in 2023 alone. Using other tracking methods, the CDC estimates that approximately 476,000 people may be diagnosed and treated for Lyme disease each year in the United States.

There is an ecological dimension to the Lyme crisis that most people have never heard about. It starts with a mouse.

The white-footed mouse is the primary reservoir for Lyme disease on the East Coast. Grey squirrels carry that role west of the Rockies. These small mammals carry the Borrelia bacteria and pass them to ticks at extraordinarily high rates. The more mice and squirrels in an area, the more infected ticks feeding on them, the more disease circulating in the environment.

The natural check on this system is the fox. Where fox populations are healthy, mouse populations stay controlled. Where foxes thrive, Lyme generally does not. The problem is that coyotes have been spreading through the Midwest and Northeast and displacing foxes. Coyotes cover more territory and hunt larger prey. They are far less effective at controlling the small rodent populations that carry Lyme. Fewer foxes means more mice. More mice means more infected ticks. More infected ticks means more sick people.

This is not a hunting or hiking problem. This is an ecosystem problem. The food web that kept tick-borne illness in check is broken. And until someone figures out how to fix that, the ticks will keep spreading.

* * *

The Bullseye Rash Myth

Here is the thing most people believe about Lyme disease: if you get it, you will see a bullseye rash.

Here is the truth: many people never get one.

The classic expanding rash, called erythema migrans, does appear in many Lyme disease cases. But the bullseye pattern is actually not as common as most people think. Studies suggest that only about 20 percent of Lyme rashes present in the classic bullseye pattern. Many appear as a solid red oval or simply as a spreading red area with no distinct rings at all. And in some patients, the rash never develops or appears in a location that is easy to miss.

Do not wait for a bullseye. If you have been outside in tick territory and you develop a rash of any kind along with flu-like symptoms, tell your doctor and ask specifically about Lyme disease.

* * *

The Chronic Lyme Controversy

Studies estimate that between 10 and 20 percent of people who are treated for Lyme disease continue to experience symptoms after completing their antibiotic course. Fatigue. Joint pain. Brain fog. Difficulty concentrating. These symptoms can persist for months or years. A recent estimate put the cumulative number of people living with Post-Treatment Lyme Disease Syndrome at close to two million in the United States.

There is also the question of sexual transmission. Some researchers have raised the possibility that Lyme disease may be transmissible through sexual contact and potentially carried to birth. The CDC says the evidence does not support this. The debate continues, and more studying is needed. If you are concerned, speak with your doctor.

Also, in rare, documented cases neurological Lyme disease has been associated with auditory hallucinations. A case report published in the Southern Medical Journal documented two patients who began hearing music that was not there. The hallucinations disappeared with IV antibiotic treatment and returned when treatment stopped. A tick bite changing someone's entire reality.

The honest answer is that the science is genuinely unresolved. What is unresolved is that real people are suffering from real symptoms and deserve to be taken seriously. If you or someone you love has been treated for Lyme disease and continues to struggle, you are not imagining it. Push for answers. Find a doctor who will listen.

* * *

The Bottom Line

Lyme disease is the most common tick-borne illness in the United States and one of the most frequently misdiagnosed. The rash you have been told to look for is only one of many ways it can present, and sometimes it does not appear at all. The tests used to diagnose it misses more than half of the cases.

If you have been in tick territory and you feel wrong, push for Lyme disease testing. If you test negative but still feel wrong, push again. The tests are not reliable enough to rule it out on the first try.

The Conspiracies

I want to be honest with you about this section before we start.

What follows is not a conspiracy theory. It is also not a settled matter. It is a collection of documented facts, credible questions, and an ongoing government investigation that, as of 2026, has not yet produced its final answers.

I am not going to tell you the government definitely created Lyme disease. I am also not going to tell you that the questions people are asking are crazy. Both of those statements would be dishonest.

What I am going to do is tell you what we know, what is documented, what has been investigated, and what is still unanswered. Then you can decide what you think.

* * *

Plum Island

Plum Island sits in the water off the eastern tip of Long Island, New York. It is a federal facility, fully owned by the United States government. It is located approximately thirteen miles from Lyme, Connecticut. The town where Lyme disease was first identified in the 1970s.

From 1952 to 1969, Plum Island was managed not by the Department of Agriculture but by the United States Army Chemical Corps, the branch responsible for biological warfare research. During that period, the facility conducted outdoor experiments with diseased ticks and maintained extensive tick breeding operations.

The Department of Agriculture has maintained that Lyme disease was never a topic of research at Plum Island. Yet, in 1993, Newsday uncovered classified documents proving that biological warfare research had in fact occurred at the facility, contradicting decades of official denials.

* * *

Willy Burgdorfer

In 1982, a Swiss-American scientist named Willy Burgdorfer identified the bacterium that causes Lyme disease. What was less publicly known was the other side of his career. He had been recruited specifically for tick-borne pathogen research and was simultaneously funded by the United States Army's biological defense program while publishing scientific papers for the public.

In 2013, journalist Kris Newby interviewed Burgdorfer on camera for a documentary. He appeared to suggest that Lyme disease was not a naturally occurring germ that had escaped into the environment but something that had come from a military bioweapons lab. Before his death in 2014, Burgdorfer left a note that read: I wondered why somebody didn't do something.

* * *

The Congressional Investigation

In late 2025, a binding investigation was enshrined in the National Defense Authorization Act for 2026. Section 1068 of that law now mandates that the Government Accountability Office conduct a full investigation, reviewing all records from 1945 through 1972 with a specific focus on tick research and the potential for environmental release.

That investigation is currently underway as this book goes to press.

* * *

What the Science Says

Research has shown that the Borrelia burgdorferi bacterium existed in North American ticks for at least 60,000 years before any government research program existed. The mainstream scientific and public health establishment attributes the dramatic rise in Lyme disease cases to reforestation of the northeastern United States, expansion of deer populations, suburban development pushing into tick habitat, and climate-driven expansion of tick ranges.

None of these explanations requires a laboratory origin. But the ancient presence of the bacterium does not rule out the possibility that laboratory activities accelerated, enhanced, or accidentally spread what was already present in nature.

* * *

What We Still Don't Know

The records from the most relevant period were largely destroyed in 1969. Willy Burgdorfer identified the Lyme pathogen, spent his career developing tick-borne bioweapons, appeared to suggest on camera that Lyme disease had laboratory origins, and then died, saying he had not told everything.

The Government Accountability Office is currently conducting its investigation. When it concludes, it may produce answers. It may produce more questions. Or it may produce a classified report that the public never sees.

Pay attention. The investigation is ongoing.

* * *

The Theories That Don't Have Full Proof Yet

The tick crisis has given rise to a number of theories that circulate online, in farming communities, and in health-conscious circles. Some of these theories are connected to documented facts. Others are based on circumstantial connections. None of them has been proven. I am not going to tell you what to believe. What I will do is present them honestly and let you decide what to do with them.

The Gates Foundation and Alpha-Gal

The Bill and Melinda Gates Foundation did fund research grants involving genetically modified ticks through a biotech company called Oxitec. The documented project focused on cattle ticks, aimed at reducing livestock disease and economic damage, and was reportedly confined to laboratory research. The tick species involved was the Asian blue tick, not the Lone Star tick, most associated with Alpha-Gal Syndrome in the United States.

Online, people connect these facts together: the Gates Foundation funded tick research. Gates has also invested heavily in alternative proteins and lab-grown meat. Alpha-Gal cases have increased, and make people allergic to red meat. Government and biotech sectors are increasingly involved in food system redesign.

That combination understandably raises suspicion for some people. What I can tell you is that the documented research involved a different species of tick than the one causing Alpha-Gal, was focused on livestock, not humans, and was reportedly confined to a laboratory. What I cannot tell you is that there is nothing else worth knowing. I don't know that. Nobody outside of those programs does.

Farmers Finding Boxes of Ticks

In the spring of 2026, a social media post from a person identifying herself as a holistic doctor claimed that farmers in the

Midwest were finding boxes of ticks on their properties. The post received tens of millions of views. NBC Chicago investigated and contacted health officials across the region. No officials confirmed any such incidents. Snopes contacted hundreds of Missouri county and city officials and found no one who could verify the claim. The person who originated the post later acknowledged she had not heard it from farmers directly but from a colleague.

As of this writing, there is no verified evidence that boxes of ticks have been found on farmland outside of TikTok videos I have come across. What I can say is that tick populations are expanding, tick season is arriving earlier, and emergency room visits for tick bites are at a nine-year high. The anxiety driving those viral posts is real, even if the specific claim has not been verified.

The Vaccine and the Crisis

It is worth noting that the most significant Lyme disease vaccine in twenty-four years is seeking FDA approval at the same moment that tick populations are at record highs, tick-borne illness cases are rising faster than at any point in recent history, and public awareness of ticks has never been greater. Pfizer stands to generate billions from a successful vaccine launch. Some people ask whether the crisis and the cure arriving together is a coincidence. That question does not have a verified answer. What is true is that fear drives demand. And demand drives profit. Make of that what you will.

Why These Theories Spread

I think about this sometimes. The government investigation into Plum Island is real. Willy Burgdorfer's dual career is real. The classified records that were destroyed are real. When people lose trust in institutions, they fill the gaps with the most alarming explanation available. I understand that impulse. I have spent my life in rooms where the official answer didn't fit what I was seeing with my own eyes.

But I also know that the difference between paying attention and going down a rabbit hole is evidence. You are allowed to ask questions. You are allowed to be skeptical. You are allowed to think the official explanation is incomplete. What I'd ask is that you hold the unverified theories loosely and follow the documented facts closely. The documented facts are alarming enough.

The Other Illnesses: What Ticks Are Carrying Beyond Lyme

By now, you know about Lyme disease, Rocky Mountain Spotted Fever, and Alpha-Gal Syndrome. But ticks are carrying more than that. Here are four more illnesses most people have never heard of and shouldn't have to find out about the hard way.

* * *

Babesiosis

Babesiosis is unlike any other tick-borne illness on this list. It is not caused by a bacterium. It is caused by a microscopic parasite called Babesia microti that infects red blood cells. The closest medical comparison is malaria.

An estimated 50 percent of infected children and 25 percent of adults show no symptoms at all. For older adults, people without a spleen, or people with weakened immune systems, it can be life-threatening.

Symptoms in those who do become ill include fever, chills, sweating, fatigue, loss of appetite, muscle aches, and headache.

Because these symptoms resemble many other illnesses, including the flu, babesiosis is frequently misdiagnosed or missed entirely. A blood smear or PCR test is needed to confirm it, and your doctor has to think about ordering it.

Babesiosis does not respond to doxycycline. It requires a different treatment. It's typically a combination of atovaquone and azithromycin for mild to moderate cases. Getting the right diagnosis matters. Not just any treatment for tick-borne illness, but the right one.

* * *

Powassan Virus

Powassan is the one on this list that should frighten you the most. It is caused by a virus, which means antibiotics do nothing against it. There is no specific treatment. There is no vaccine. Approximately ten percent of people who develop the severe neurological form of the disease die from it. More than half of survivors experience long-term neurological problems.

Symptoms appear one week to one month after the bite of an infected tick. Early symptoms include fever, headache, vomiting, and weakness. As the disease progresses, it can cause confusion, loss of coordination, difficulty speaking, and seizures. In severe cases, it can cause encephalitis (inflammation of the brain) and meningitis. Survivors often experience long-term neurological problems, including recurring headaches and memory loss.

Most tick-borne diseases require a tick to be attached for 24 to 48 hours before transmission can occur. The Powassan virus can be transmitted in as little as 15 minutes after a tick attaches. You may never even know the tick was there.

* * *

Ehrlichiosis

Ehrlichiosis is caused by bacteria in the Ehrlichia family and is transmitted primarily by the Lone Star tick. Symptoms are nearly identical to anaplasmosis: fever, headache, muscle aches, fatigue. Severe cases can involve respiratory failure, bleeding problems, kidney failure, and neurological complications. Like anaplasmosis, it responds to doxycycline when treated promptly.

Symptoms typically appear five to fourteen days after a tick bite and include fever, chills, severe headache, muscle aches, fatigue, and sometimes nausea and vomiting. A rash appears in some cases but not all. If untreated, the disease can progress to severe illness, including respiratory failure, kidney failure, and neurological complications. Like anaplasmosis, it responds well to doxycycline when caught early, but your doctor has to think to test for it.

* * *

Anaplasmosis

Anaplasmosis is caused by a bacterium called Anaplasma phagocytophilum, transmitted primarily by blacklegged ticks. Symptoms typically appear one to two weeks after a tick bite: fever, chills, severe headache, muscle aches, and fatigue. A rash is present in fewer than ten percent of cases. About 32 percent of anaplasmosis cases in Minnesota require hospitalization. It responds well to doxycycline when caught early.

A woman in her forties in Puyallup, Washington, was hospitalized for 10 days after being bitten by an infected tick in the brushy areas around Puyallup and Eatonville. She was fortunate they found it, and she recovered. Wherever you live, ticks are moving closer.

Ticks are not only threatening humans. A disease called Bobcat Fever is clinically known as Cytauxzoonosis and is spreading rapidly across the United States. Transmitted primarily by the Lone Star tick, Bobcat Fever has a death rate of 97 percent in untreated cats and can kill within 48 hours of symptoms appearing. Cases are rising as tick populations expand northward and southward simultaneously. If you have an outdoor cat, talk to your veterinarian about tick prevention immediately. One bite from the wrong tick can be a death sentence.

Infected cats develop high fever, lethargy, and loss of appetite rapidly. Without immediate veterinary treatment, most do not survive.

* * *

The Bigger Picture

A single tick can carry more than one of these pathogens simultaneously. A patient who tests negative for Lyme disease may still have anaplasmosis or babesiosis. The message from every illness in this book is the same: if you have been outside and you develop a sudden fever with headache and body aches, tell your doctor. Mention ticks. Ask about tick-borne illness specifically.

You are the one who knows something is off. Don't brush it off.

Where Ticks Hide

The first thing most people think of when they hear about tick-borne illness is hiking. Deep woods. Tall grass. Wilderness trails far from civilization.

My husband got five ticks on his back from walking a paved path on a beautiful afternoon.

Ticks are not waiting for you to do something adventurous. They are waiting in your backyard, in the grass along your fence line, in the leaf pile your kids jumped in last weekend, and on the deer that walked through your neighborhood at dawn.

* * *

Where Ticks Live: The Environment

Ticks do not jump, fly, or fall from trees. They find their hosts through a behavior called questing, which means they climb to the tip of a blade of grass, a leaf, or a low branch and hold on with their back legs while reaching their front legs out, waiting to grab onto anything that brushes past. They thrive in humid environments and are almost always found low to the ground, rarely higher than about three feet.

What researchers have recently discovered makes this even more unsettling. A 2023 study published in Current Biology found that ticks may not even need to make direct contact with you. The naturally occurring static electricity that humans and animals accumulate as they move through the world is enough to pull a tick across an air gap several times larger than its own body, launching it onto a host it never physically touched. One researcher described it as the equivalent of a person jumping three or four flights of stairs in a single leap. You do not have to brush against the grass. You just have to walk near it.

Your yard is not automatically safe. Any area where wildlife passes through can bring ticks onto your property. A deer walking through your yard at night leaves behind ticks that drop off and begin seeking new hosts in your grass by morning.

People often say ticks are becoming more aggressive. What they are really seeing is more ticks in more places at more times of year.

Emergency room visits for tick bites were up 25 percent in April 2026 over the same month the year before. Tick populations in some areas increased by 145 percent in a single year. Species like the Lone Star tick are now showing up in states where they were almost never found before. The ticks are not coming for you. There are just more of them, and they are spreading.

* * *

Where Ticks Hide on Your Body

The places most commonly missed during tick checks include the scalp and hairline, behind and inside the ears, the back of the neck, under the arms and in the armpits, around and inside the belly button, in the groin and between the legs, behind the knees, and between the toes.

After every outdoor activity, even a walk on a paved path, do a full body check on yourself, your children, and your pets. Use a mirror for hard-to-see areas. Run your fingers through your hair.

Ticks find the places you are not looking. That is the whole lesson.

How to Repel Ticks

No repellent is perfect. No strategy eliminates the risk entirely. But the right combination of tools can dramatically reduce your chances of a tick ever finding you.

* * *

Permethrin: The Most Powerful Tool You Have

If you only do one thing after reading this section, treat your clothing with permethrin. Unlike skin repellents that mask your scent, permethrin attacks a tick's nervous system the moment it touches treated fabric. Ticks that crawl across permethrin-treated clothing don't just turn around and leave. They die.

Research from the University of Rhode Island found that people wearing permethrin-treated shoes and socks were 73.6 times less likely to be bitten by a tick than those wearing untreated footwear.

One important warning: Permethrin is toxic to cats. Do not use it on or near cats, and keep treated clothing away from them until it is fully dry.

The good news is that you do not need to apply permethrin to your skin. It is applied to your clothing and gear, your pants, shirt, socks, and boots before you head out. You can treat your own clothing at home with a spray like Repel Permethrin, available at REI, Dick's Sporting Goods, Walmart, and Amazon. One treatment lasts through several washes. If you would rather skip the spraying entirely, companies like Insect Shield sell pre-treated clothing that is factory-treated and lasts up to 70 washes. It is worth the investment if you spend regular time outdoors. Let it be noted that it can be messy if you apply it yourself.

* * *

DEET — The Gold Standard for Skin

DEET has been used since 1946 and remains the most well-researched skin repellent available. The CDC recommends products containing DEET concentrations between 20 and 30 percent for optimal protection against ticks. Higher concentrations do not repel better; they just last slightly longer.

One important warning: Permethrin is toxic to children 3 and under and to cats. Do not use it on or near cats, and keep treated clothing away from them until it is fully dry.

* * *

Natural Options: What Works and What Doesn't

Oil of Lemon Eucalyptus, also called OLE, is the one natural option that the CDC recognizes as effective. It provides meaningful protection comparable to lower concentrations of DEET, roughly four to six hours of protection per application. Important note: Do not use OLE on children under three years old.

Essential oils like citronella, peppermint, cedar oil, and lavender are frequently recommended online, but the scientific evidence for these options against ticks is limited and inconsistent. If you choose essential oil-based repellents, pairing them with permethrin-treated clothing has been proven to work well.

* * *

After You Come In

Shower within two hours of coming in from tick territory. Do a thorough check of yourself, your children, and your pets. Tumble dry your clothes in a dryer on high heat for ten minutes to kill any remaining ticks.

And if you find one, go to the next section.

How to Remove a Tick Safely

You found one. Take a breath. You have time to do this right.

Most tick-borne diseases require a tick to be attached for at least 24 to 36 hours before transmission can occur. Finding a tick early and removing it promptly and correctly significantly reduces your risk. The keyword is correctly. Because there is a lot of folk wisdom out there about tick removal that is not just unhelpful but actively makes things worse.

* * *

The Right Way: Step by Step

Step one: Get as close to the skin as possible with fine-tipped pointed tweezers. Grip the tick as close to where it has attached as you can.

Step two: Pull upward with steady, even pressure. Do not twist. Do not jerk. A slow, steady upward pull is what you want.

Step three: If the mouthparts break off and stay in the skin, try to remove them. If you cannot get them out easily, leave them and let the skin heal.

Step four: Clean the bite area and your hands thoroughly with rubbing alcohol, iodine, or soap and water.

Step four and a half: Apply a topical antibiotic ointment such as bacitracin or Polysporin to the bite site. Reapply daily for a few days while it heals. This treats the bite wound the same way you would treat any other minor skin wound. It does not prevent disease, but it protects against local infection at the site and is specifically recommended after tick removal.

Step five: Save the tick. Place it in a sealed plastic bag with the date and location written on the outside. Even a dead tick can be identified by species and, in some cases, tested for pathogens.

Step six: Dispose of the tick by putting the sealed bag in the trash or submitting it to your local health department for identification.

* * *

What NOT to Do

Do not use a lit match or a lighter. Applying heat to a tick can cause it to release saliva or regurgitate stomach contents into the wound. I grew up watching ticks removed from animals this way. The research is now detailed enough that it causes more harm than good.

Do not coat the tick with petroleum jelly, Vaseline, alcohol, or nail polish. Do not twist the tick as you pull. Do not squeeze or crush the tick's body, and do not remove the tick with your bare fingers.

* * *

After Removal: What to Watch For

Watch the bite site and your overall health for the next month. If anything feels off: fever, fatigue, a rash, a headache that doesn't feel like your normal headache. Don't wait it out. The section below breaks down exactly what to watch for and why timing matters so much.

* * *

Signs Something Is Wrong

Emergency room visits for tick bites in 2026 are the highest they have been since 2017. Most people who get bitten by a tick will not get sick. But some will. And the difference between a full recovery and a serious illness is almost always the same thing: how quickly someone recognized that something was wrong and got the right treatment.

Fever appearing within one to four weeks of a tick bite is the most important warning sign across all tick-borne illnesses. Severe headache, especially one that comes on suddenly and feels different from a normal headache. Fatigue that is not explained by activity level or sleep. Muscle and joint aches that appear without explanation. Any rash, especially one that appears near a tick bite or that expands over time.

The bottom line: if you feel like you have the flu within a month of a tick bite, tell your doctor about the bite. Do not assume it is just a virus. Make them consider tick-borne illness.

* * *

Lyme Disease — Symptoms appear 3 to 30 days after bite

Early Lyme disease often feels like the flu. Fever, chills, headache, fatigue, muscle and joint aches, and swollen lymph nodes. About 60 percent of people with Lyme disease develop a rash, but only about 20 percent of those rashes have the classic bullseye pattern.

* * *

Rocky Mountain Spotted Fever — Symptoms appear 2 to 14 days after bite

RMSF comes on fast and hard. High fever, often above 102 or 103 degrees, severe headache, nausea and vomiting, muscle pain, and sensitivity to light. This disease moves fast. Without treatment, death can occur within eight days of symptoms beginning. If you or someone you love develops a sudden high fever with a severe headache after tick exposure, do not wait. Go to the doctor that day.

I know this one personally. The doctors gave me one day to live. Early treatment is everything.

* * *

Powassan Virus — Symptoms appear 1 week to 1 month after bite

There is no specific treatment for Powassan. If someone develops neurological symptoms, including confusion, loss of coordination, or seizures after tick exposure, this is a medical emergency. Go to the emergency room immediately. Powassan can be transmitted in as little as 15 minutes after a tick attaches.

* * *

Alpha-Gal Syndrome — Symptoms appear 3 to 6 hours after eating red meat

Alpha-Gal Syndrome is different from every other illness on this list because the symptoms don't appear after the tick bite. They appear hours after eating red meat, sometimes weeks or months after the bite that caused the sensitization. If you develop unexplained allergic reactions hours after eating red meat, ask your doctor specifically about Alpha-Gal Syndrome. Forty-two percent of doctors have never heard of it. You may have to be the one who brings it up.

* * *

What to Say to Your Doctor

Tell them you were bitten by a tick or spent time outdoors in tick territory. Tell them the date of the bite if you know it. Bring the tick if you saved it. Ask specifically: could this be a tick-borne illness? Ask about testing. Ask about whether to start doxycycline while waiting for results.

If your doctor dismisses your concern without adequate explanation, you have the right to ask more questions or seek a second opinion. You know your body. Trust it.

What Is Coming: The Race for a Tick Vaccine

For most of this book, I have been telling you what ticks are carrying right now and what to do about it. I touched on the vaccine briefly earlier, but it deserves its own space. Before I close, I want to tell you what is on the horizon. Because something significant is happening and you deserve to know about it. The Lyme disease vaccine is closer than it has ever been.

The History You Should Know

There was a Lyme disease vaccine before. Most people have forgotten that or never knew it.

In 1998, the FDA approved LYMErix, a vaccine developed by SmithKline Beecham. It was the first and only Lyme disease vaccine ever approved for human use. Clinical trials showed it was about 76 to 92 percent effective after three doses. It worked.

And then it didn't exist anymore.

What happened was not a safety failure. The vaccine was pulled from the market in 2002 after a public backlash driven largely by unfounded concerns that it might cause arthritis. The studies did not support that conclusion. Regulatory bodies and independent researchers reviewed the data and found no credible evidence of harm. But the lawsuits, the media coverage, and the drop in demand made it commercially unviable. SmithKline Beecham quietly discontinued it.

The Lyme disease community has been living without a vaccine ever since. For twenty-four years.

* * *

VLA15: The Vaccine in Phase 3

In March 2026, Pfizer and their partner Valneva announced the topline results from their Phase 3 VALOR trial, which stands for Vaccine Against Lyme for Outdoor Recreationists, and the results were significant. The investigational vaccine, now designated PF-07307405, demonstrated 73.2 percent efficacy in reducing confirmed Lyme disease cases in participants aged five and older. It was well tolerated. No serious safety concerns were identified. Pfizer is now preparing to submit a Biologics License Application to the FDA. If approved, this would be the first Lyme disease vaccine available to the public in over two decades.

The trial enrolled more than 9,400 participants across the United States, Canada, and Europe in areas where Lyme disease is highly endemic. Participants received three doses in the primary series, followed by a booster dose before the next tick season. The trial tracked actual Lyme disease cases, not just immune response measurements, which makes the 73 percent efficacy figure meaningful in real-world terms.

* * *

What This Vaccine Does and Does Not Do

This is where I want you to pay very close attention, because a Lyme vaccine being approved would be genuinely wonderful news and also not the end of the tick crisis.

What it does: It targets Lyme disease specifically. If approved and if the efficacy holds, it would meaningfully reduce the risk of contracting Borrelia burgdorferi, the most common tick-borne pathogen in the United States. For families in endemic areas, that is significant protection.

What it does not do: It does not protect against any of the other tick-borne illnesses covered in this book. Not Rocky Mountain Spotted Fever. Not Alpha-Gal Syndrome. Not anaplasmosis, ehrlichiosis, babesiosis, or Powassan virus. A vaccinated person who gets bitten by a tick can still develop any of those conditions.

There is no vaccine for RMSF. There is no vaccine for Alpha-Gal Syndrome. There is no vaccine for the Powassan virus, which is transmitted in as little as fifteen minutes and has no treatment. Vaccines for those illnesses are in various early stages of research, but none are close to the market.

A Lyme vaccine is not a solution to the tick crisis. It is a meaningful piece of one. The prevention measures in this book still matter. Tick checks still matter. Knowing the warning signs still matters. Knowing what to say to your doctor still matters.

* * *

The Earlier Vaccine and Why It Matters

I think about LYMErix sometimes. I think about the families who could have been protected between 2002 and now. The people who got Lyme disease during those twenty-four years, who developed Post-Treatment Lyme Disease Syndrome, whose lives changed in ways that did not have to happen if a safe and effective vaccine had stayed on the market.

I also think about what pulled it off the market. Not evidence. Not science. Public pressure driven by fear and misinformation, amplified faster than the facts could keep up. And a company that decided the commercial risk wasn't worth it. Maybe it worked? You know what people say about vaccines these days.

I am not going to tell you what to think about vaccines. That is not my place, and it is not what this book is about. Just be sure to do your homework. What I will tell you is that if a Lyme vaccine is approved and your doctor recommends it for your family, the decision deserves to be made based on the actual clinical data, not on what happened in 1998, not on fear, and not on things you read without a source attached.

My grandmother made a decision based on what she read in a magazine. She read carefully. She connected dots. She acted on the evidence. That is what I am asking you to do, too.

* * *

What to Ask Your Doctor

If a Lyme vaccine is approved by the time this book is in your hands, here is what to ask your physician:

Am I or is my family in a high-risk area for Lyme disease? Is this vaccine recommended for my age group? How many doses are required and when? Does it require an annual booster? Does my insurance cover it? And importantly, what tick-borne illnesses am I still at risk for even if I am vaccinated?

That last question is the one most people will not think to ask. Now you will.

A vaccine against Lyme disease is not permission to stop checking yourself after you come inside. It is not a reason to skip the tick check on your children or your pets. Ticks carry more than Lyme disease and always have. My grandmother was not reading about

Lyme disease that summer in Florida. She was reading about Rocky Mountain Spotted Fever. The ticks that nearly killed my brother and me were not carrying Borrelia burgdorferi.

Tick awareness is not a Lyme disease problem. It is a tick problem. And a vaccine for one illness, however welcome, does not change that.

* * *

In May 2026, Health Secretary Robert F. Kennedy Jr. announced millions of dollars in funding for Lyme disease research. The Department of Health and Human Services committed up to $2 million to AI-driven projects helping patients get answers faster and announced three new LymeX innovation challenges with up to $2.5 million in total prize funding. The government is paying attention. The question is whether it is fast enough.

Beverly, my grandma would have loved this news. She read everything. She paid attention to things. She would have found the article about the Phase 3 results, and she would have talked about it at the kitchen table while smoking her cigarette and drinking her coffee.

If she were alive today she undoubtably would have told you to check for ticks when you came inside. Some things do not change.

Don't Brush It Off

I wrote this book for you.

Not the version of you that has everything figured out. The version of you that is sitting in a waiting room, wondering if you are overreacting. The version of you that just found something on your child's scalp and your heart is in your throat. The version of you that knows something is wrong with someone you love and has been told so many times to relax, to wait and see, to stop catastrophizing, that you have started to believe them.

I wrote this for the person who is not sure they know anything at all but knows they need to say something anyway.

That person has saved more lives than any doctor I have ever met.

* * *

My grandmother was not a medical professional. She was a woman sitting at home reading a magazine. She read something and something in her lit up and said this is it. And instead of talking herself out of it, instead of worrying that she would look foolish or like an alarmist or that the doctors would dismiss her, she brought that magazine to the hospital and waited for the doctor to arrive.

She was the crazy lady in the room that day.

She saved our lives.

I have spent my whole life paying attention. Not because I always know what I am talking about. I do not. Not because I am never wrong. I am. But because paying attention and speaking up, even when you are not sure, even when you are afraid of being dismissed, is the most important thing I know how to do.

* * *

There are threats everywhere in life. Ticks in the grass on a beautiful afternoon. Symptoms that look like a hundred other things. Doctors are overworked and undertrained in the very conditions that are becoming more common every year.

You cannot eliminate the threats. None of us can. What you can do is refuse to let them cripple you. Let them make you more present. More observant. More willing to speak up in the rooms where you are afraid of being the one who is wrong.

The worst thing that happens when you speak up, and you are wrong is that it stings for a second and then everyone moves on. However, the worst thing that happens when you stay quiet, and you were right, is something you or someone else may never recover from.

Speak up. Every time. Don't brush it off.

* * *

I want to tell you one more thing before I let you go.

There will be moments when you speak up, and nothing comes of it. When the tests come back clear, and the doctor looks at you with that particular expression that means we are done here, and you walk out of the office feeling foolish. There will be moments when you push and push, and the answer you find is not the dramatic answer you were afraid of, just something ordinary and easily fixed. Those moments will make you want to stop pushing.

Don't let them.

Every time I have been wrong, I have been relieved. Relief is the correct response to being wrong. Being wrong means nothing terrible is happening. It means you can go home and exhale and have dinner with your family and wake up the next morning with everything still intact. I have never once been wrong and wished I had stayed quiet. I have been wrong and still called it a good day.

Being right when something is wrong is not the goal. The goal is paying attention consistently enough that when something is wrong, you catch it. And the only way to do that is to keep the habit going even when it turns up nothing. Even when it turns up nothing a hundred times in a row.

My grandmother read magazines for years. Decades. She probably never imagined she would use any of the information in them. And then one summer in Florida, her grandchildren were dying, her natural knack for making connections delivered, and she found the answer.

You don't know which thing you are paying attention to right now that will matter later. You just keep paying attention.

Write it down. Speak up. Don't wait.

That is the whole book in seven words. Everything else is the story of how I learned it.

I hope you never need any of it. I genuinely, from the bottom of my heart, hope that you read this book and put it down and never think about it again because nothing in your life ever requires you to fight for an answer in a hospital room.

But if you do need it, I hope it is there for you. I hope you hear my grandmother's voice and mine, and every person in this book who paid attention and spoke up, even when they were not sure.

I hope you feel less alone in that room. I hope you say the thing.

That is why I wrote it. That is the whole reason.

* * *

Be the crazy lady in the room. I promise you, you are already her. You have been reading a book about ticks and pituitary tumors, and government conspiracies, because something in you said to pay attention. That instinct is a gift.

Don't brush it off.

Tick Identification Guide

SIZE REFERENCE

Ticks are small. Most people never see them until they are already attached.

Poppy Seed — Nymph. Most dangerous. Hardest to see.

Sesame Seed — Unfed adult tick. Most common find.

Watermelon Seed — Larger species, unfed. American and Rocky Mountain Wood tick.

Raisin to Grape — Engorged and fully fed. Has been attached for hours or days.

COMMON TICKS IN THE UNITED STATES

Blacklegged / Deer Tick — Sesame seed size. Orange-brown body, dark legs, no markings. *Carries: Lyme disease, anaplasmosis, babesiosis, Powassan virus*

American Dog Tick — Watermelon seed size. Brown with white and gray streaks on the back. *Carries: Rocky Mountain Spotted Fever, tularemia*

Lone Star Tick — Sesame seed size. Reddish-brown with a single white spot on the female. *Carries: Alpha-Gal Syndrome, ehrlichiosis, tularemia*

Rocky Mountain Wood Tick — Watermelon seed size. Brown with white-gray markings on the back. *Carries: Rocky Mountain Spotted Fever, Colorado tick fever*

Brown Dog Tick — Sesame seed size. Reddish-brown, no markings. *Carries: Rocky Mountain Spotted Fever*

Western Blacklegged Tick — Sesame seed size. Orange-brown body, dark legs. *Carries: Lyme disease, anaplasmosis*

Tick ranges are expanding. If you spend time outdoors anywhere in the United States, ticks are a risk.

WHERE TICKS LIVE IN THE UNITED STATES

Ticks are found in every state. The following shows primary concentration areas — not hard borders.

Northeast — Blacklegged/Deer Tick — Lyme disease, anaplasmosis, babesiosis, Powassan virus

Upper Midwest — Blacklegged/Deer Tick — Lyme disease, anaplasmosis, babesiosis

Southeast — Lone Star Tick, American Dog Tick — Alpha-Gal Syndrome, RMSF, ehrlichiosis

South Central — Lone Star Tick — Alpha-Gal Syndrome, ehrlichiosis, tularemia

Rocky Mountains — Rocky Mountain Wood Tick, Dog Tick — RMSF, Colorado tick fever

Pacific Coast — Western Blacklegged Tick — Lyme disease, anaplasmosis

All 48 States — Brown Dog Tick — Rocky Mountain Spotted Fever

Note: The Brown Dog Tick is found in all 48 contiguous states, including indoors and in kennels. Alaska and Hawaii have their own tick species and risks. Consult your local health department.

AFTER A TICK BITE — QUICK REFERENCE

Use fine-tipped tweezers. Grip as close to the skin as possible. Pull straight up with steady pressure. Do not twist.

Clean the bite area. Use rubbing alcohol, iodine, or soap and water.

Apply bacitracin or Polysporin. Reapply daily for a few days while it heals.

Save the tick. Sealed plastic bag. Write the date and location. It can be identified or tested.

Watch for symptoms for 30 days. Fever, headache, rash, fatigue, and muscle aches. Call your doctor if any appear.

Do NOT use heat, petroleum jelly, or nail polish to remove a tick.

CALL YOUR DOCTOR IMMEDIATELY IF YOU HAVE:

High Fever + Severe Headache — Especially within 14 days of a bite. Could be RMSF. Do not wait.

Any Rash — With or without the classic bullseye. Rashes appear in many forms.

Confusion or Neurological Symptoms — Seizures, loss of coordination. Possible Powassan virus. Go to the ER.

Allergic Reaction After Red Meat — Hours after eating, not minutes. Ask about Alpha-Gal Syndrome specifically.

Flu-Like Symptoms — Within a month of outdoor activity. Mention ticks to your doctor.

Rapid Swelling at Bite Site — Or difficulty breathing. Seek emergency care immediately.

Don't Brush It Off. jennifersaterdal.com

Resources and Sources

Government and Public Health Centers for Disease Control and Prevention — cdc.gov/ticks National Defense Authorization Act for Fiscal Year 2026 — Section 1068

Clinical Research Clinical Infectious Diseases Journal — RMSF long-term complications study IDSA 2020 Guidelines — Babesiosis diagnosis and management American College of Gastroenterology — Alpha-gal antibody study November 2025 University of Rhode Island — Permethrin effectiveness research Current Biology Journal — Static electricity and tick transmission 2023 Stricker RB, Winger EE. Musical Hallucinations in Patients with Lyme Disease. Southern Medical Journal. 2003;96(7):711-715 American Psychological Association — Lyme disease and neuropsychiatric symptoms — apa.org 2022 Journal of Allergy and Clinical Immunology: In Practice — First documented Alpha-Gal fatality — November 2025 University of Virginia School of Medicine — Alpha-Gal Syndrome death case study — November 2025

Vaccine Research Pfizer and Valneva — Phase 3 VALOR Trial — March 2026 LYMErix — FDA approval 1998 and market withdrawal 2002 HHS — LymeX Innovation Challenges and Lyme funding announcement May 2026

Books Newby, Kris. Bitten: The Secret History of Lyme Disease and Biological Weapons. Harper Wave, 2019.

Journalism McDonald, John. "Plum Island's Shadowy Past." Newsday, November 21, 1993 NBC Chicago — Boxes of ticks investigation spring 2026 Snopes — Boxes of ticks fact-check — snopes.com Snopes — Gates Foundation tick research fact-check — snopes.com Politifact — Gates Foundation Oxitec tick research fact-check — politifact.com

Tick Repellent Products Insect Shield — insectshield.com Repel Permethrin — Available at REI, Dick's Sporting Goods, Walmart, Amazon

Organizations LymeDisease.org — lymedisease.org Bay Area Lyme Foundation — bayarealyme.org Global Lyme Alliance — globallymealliance.org Generation Lyme — genlyme.org Tick Encounter Resource Center — tickencounter.org

About the Author

Jennifer Saterdal is a mom, grandmother, tick illness survivor, and author from Puyallup, Washington. At age eight, she and her brother were given one and two days to live from Rocky Mountain Spotted Fever. Her grandmother saved their lives by recognizing their symptoms from a magazine article when the hospital had run out of answers. That experience shaped everything about how Jennifer pays attention to the people she loves.

As an outdoor enthusiast who loves hiking and camping, Jennifer knows firsthand that ticks don't wait for you to do something dramatic. They are just there. On the trail. In the grass. Anywhere on a beautiful afternoon.

She is the author of *Bitten: A Tick Survivor's Warning About the Growing Tick Crisis*, published under her imprint Don't Brush It Off Publishing, an imprint of NextJen LLC. She writes and advocates for tick awareness because she believes the information in this book could save lives.

Jennifer lives in Puyallup, Washington, with her family.

jennifersaterdal.com

www.ingramcontent.com/pod-product-compliance
Lightning Source LLC
LaVergne TN
LVHW090330210926
848480LV00004B/1356
9798988152002